T0321180

Cambridge Elements ☰

Elements of Improving Quality and Safety in Healthcare
edited by
Mary Dixon-Woods,* Katrina Brown,* Sonja Marjanovic,†
Tom Ling,† Ellen Perry,* and Graham Martin*
*THIS Institute (The Healthcare Improvement Studies Institute)
†RAND Europe

APPROACHES TO SPREAD, SCALE-UP, AND SUSTAINABILITY

Chrysanthi Papoutsi,[1] Trisha Greenhalgh,[1]
and Sonja Marjanovic[2]

[1]Nuffield Department of Primary Care Health Services, University of Oxford
[2]RAND Europe

THIS.Institute The Healthcare Improvement Studies Institute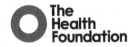

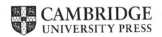
CAMBRIDGE
UNIVERSITY PRESS

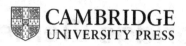

Shaftesbury Road, Cambridge CB2 8EA, United Kingdom

One Liberty Plaza, 20th Floor, New York, NY 10006, USA

477 Williamstown Road, Port Melbourne, VIC 3207, Australia

314–321, 3rd Floor, Plot 3, Splendor Forum, Jasola District Centre,
New Delhi – 110025, India

103 Penang Road, #05–06/07, Visioncrest Commercial, Singapore 238467

Cambridge University Press is part of Cambridge University Press & Assessment,
a department of the University of Cambridge.

We share the University's mission to contribute to society through the pursuit of
education, learning and research at the highest international levels of excellence.

www.cambridge.org
Information on this title: www.cambridge.org/9781009462617

DOI: 10.1017/9781009326049

First published 2024

A catalogue record for this publication is available from the British Library.

ISBN 978-1-009-46261-7 Hardback
ISBN 978-1-009-32603-2 Paperback
ISSN 2754-2912 (online)
ISSN 2754-2904 (print)

Cambridge University Press & Assessment has no responsibility for the persistence
or accuracy of URLs for external or third-party internet websites referred to in this
publication and does not guarantee that any content on such websites is, or will
remain, accurate or appropriate.

Every effort has been made in preparing this Element to provide accurate and up-to-date information
that is in accord with accepted standards and practice at the time of publication. Although case
histories are drawn from actual cases, every effort has been made to disguise the identities of the
individuals involved. Nevertheless, the authors, editors, and publishers can make no warranties that
the information contained herein is totally free from error, not least because clinical standards are
constantly changing through research and regulation. The authors, editors, and publishers therefore
disclaim all liability for direct or consequential damages resulting from the use of material contained
in this Element. Readers are strongly advised to pay careful attention to information provided by the
manufacturer of any drugs or equipment that they plan to use.

Approaches to Spread, Scale-Up, and Sustainability

Elements of Improving Quality and Safety in Healthcare

DOI: 10.1017/9781009326049
First published online: January 2024

Chrysanthi Papoutsi,[1] Trisha Greenhalgh,[1] and Sonja Marjanovic[2]
[1]*Nuffield Department of Primary Care Health Services, University of Oxford*
[2]*RAND Europe*

Author for correspondence: Chrysanthi Papoutsi,
chrysanthi.papoutsi@phc.ox.ac.uk

Abstract: Few interventions that succeed in improving healthcare locally end up becoming spread and sustained more widely. This indicates that we need to think differently about spreading improvements in practice. Drawing on a focused review of academic and grey literature, the authors outline how spread, scale-up, and sustainability have been defined and operationalised, highlighting areas of ambiguity and contention. Following an overview of relevant frameworks and models, they focus on three specific approaches and unpack their theoretical assumptions and practical implications: the Dynamic Sustainability Framework, the 3S (structure, strategy, supports) infrastructure approach for scale-up, and the NASSS (non-adoption, abandonment, and challenges to scale-up, spread, and sustainability) framework. Key points are illustrated through empirical case narratives and the Element concludes with actionable learning for those engaged in improvement activities and for researchers. This title is also available as Open Access on Cambridge Core.

Keywords: spread, scale-up, sustainability, infrastructure, adoption

ISBNs: 9781009462617 (HB), 9781009326032 (PB), 9781009326049 (OC)
ISSNs: 2754-2912 (online), 2754-2904 (print)

Contents

1 Introduction

Spread, scale-up, and sustainability are long-standing priorities for those seeking improvement in their services, as well as researchers and policymakers. In the UK, several policy programmes emphasise the need to successfully embed improvements across settings, while recognising that this can be fraught with challenges.[1–3] Other countries also put significant effort into spreading proven clinical and population health interventions – both at a national level, as in the USA[4] and Australia,[5] and at a global level, with a view to strengthening health systems across low-income and middle-income countries.[6,7]

Despite much ambition and enthusiasm, few improvement efforts that succeed locally end up being spread and sustained more widely.[8–10] In part, this may be due to the dominance of linear and prescriptive ways of conceptualising and pursuing spread, scale-up, and sustainability. By focusing primarily on short-term outcomes in a small set of contexts, improvement efforts have sometimes neglected learning from complex organisational and system-level innovations that unfold over time.[11] Spread is largely studied as the sum of multiple implementations rather than as a phenomenon in its own right.[12] And discussion of how different types of improvement efforts may require different approaches to spread, scale-up, and sustainability has been limited.

We need to think differently about spreading improvement in practice. At the time of writing, the stability of health systems has been challenged by the COVID-19 pandemic, which has compounded pre-existing system stressors, such as rising rates of long-term conditions, ageing populations, dwindling financial resources, a workforce under pressure, and the emergence of expensive investigations, technologies, and therapies. Improving the capacity and capability to better understand, plan, and operationalise spread, scale-up, and sustainability could help to reduce waste and support more focused efforts to improve health outcomes consistently and equitably.[13]

This Element begins by examining approaches to spread, scale-up, and sustainability of improvements and innovations (for brevity, we will primarily use the term 'improvements' to refer to both). We consider improvements and innovations to involve novel sets of behaviours, tools, routines, and ways of working (technological or not) that are directed at improving health and service outcomes, efficiency, effectiveness, or experience.[14] We provide an overview of different models and frameworks, before discussing three examples in more detail:

- the Dynamic Sustainability Framework[15]
- the 3S scale-up infrastructure approach[16]

- the NASSS (non-adoption, abandonment, and challenges to scale-up, spread, and sustainability) framework.[8]

To varying degrees, these three examples foreground spread, scale-up, and sustainability as adaptive processes in complex systems characterised by uncertainty, unpredictability, and emergence (i.e. when new properties arise from interactions within the system). We present the strengths and limitations of each and highlight their theoretical and applied import. Using empirical case studies, we discuss how different ways of viewing spread and scale-up make a difference in practice. At the end of the Element we distil key practical lessons to support improvement practitioners and researchers in developing sustainable and scalable improvement initiatives and interventions.

2 Spread, Scale-Up, and Sustainability in the Context of Healthcare Improvement

2.1 What Are Spread, Scale-Up, and Sustainability?

Although a growing literature discusses spread, scale-up, and sustainability in the context of healthcare improvement and innovation,[3,17–21] not all studies provide operational definitions, and some use the terms interchangeably to broadly describe implementation beyond the setting where improvement originally occurred or the intervention was piloted.

Where definitions are provided, they typically distinguish between spread as the adoption of new ways of working by new users, and scale-up as the extent to which the improvement initiative is adopted more widely within a sector (e.g. see definitions in Albury et al.[22]). What sets the two constructs apart is not so much the processes followed, as the expected end result in terms of scope and coverage.[23] Spread has been used to refer to replication of the original improvement initiative elsewhere, with or without modification.[23,24] Scale-up is assumed to involve both breadth and depth, in that improvement initiatives are reaching new users while also sustaining their presence with existing adopters, usually at organisational level.[25] Côté-Boileau et al. provide a definition of scale as 'the ambition or process of expanding the coverage of health interventions' but also refer to 'increasing the financial, human and capital resources required to expand coverage'.[23]

Operational definitions of sustainability broadly centre around whether the improvement programme (or some of its components) continues to exist in the longer term in the original setting.[26] Braithwaite et al. conceptualise sustainability as 'the continuation of programme or programme components, or the continuation of outcomes, after initial implementation efforts, staff training or funding has ended'.[13] The National Health Service (NHS) Sustainability Model adopts a view of sustainability more akin to normalisation where 'new ways of working and improved outcomes become the norm' without reverting to previous practices.[27] Drawing on a review of published literature, Moore et al. combine five constructs in their definition:

> (1) after a defined period of time, (2) the program, clinical intervention, and/ or implementation strategies continue to be delivered and/or (3) individual behaviour change (i.e. clinician, patient) is maintained; (4) the program and individual behaviour change may evolve or adapt while (5) continuing to produce benefits for individuals/systems.[28]

Sensitised by how the three constructs have been discussed in the literature, we lay out in Box 1 the definitions of spread, scale-up, and sustainability that we use in this Element.

A range of other terms have been used to describe widespread implementation, including: diffusion (passive social influence that leads to adoption), dissemination (active and planned efforts towards adoption), replication (adopting the same intervention elsewhere), continuation, durability, mainstreaming, routinisation, standardisation, institutionalisation, maintenance, and normalisation, for example, see Braithwaite et al.,[13] Côté-Boileau et al.,[23] and Greenhalgh.[29] There have been calls to improve definitional consistency and enhance practical application,[30] but the range of disciplines and theoretical orientations contributing to scholarly and applied discussions on spread, scale-up, and sustainability would make it difficult to reach consensus.[14]

Nevertheless, the terms and language we use to describe these processes denote assumptions about how we expect spread, scale-up, and sustainability to take place. This can have real consequences for the way we study and operationalise spread, scale-up, and sustainability. For example, assumptions hidden behind terminology manifest strongly in earlier traditions on the diffusion of innovations: value-laden (and persistent) terms such as 'early adopters' or 'laggards' were common. Rather than acknowledge or emphasise the influence

---

BOX 1 DEFINITIONS OF SPREAD, SCALE-UP, AND SUSTAINABILITY

In this Element, we will use terms as follows:[8,17]

- Spread: transferring successful improvement interventions beyond the original adoption setting.
- Scale-up: developing infrastructure to underpin and support widespread implementation of improvement interventions.
- Sustainability: maintaining improvements (through adaptation to context) over time.

of contextual factors, such terms created an impression that adoption is largely a matter of user willingness to follow a relatively smooth, predetermined route of engaging with innovations seen as inherently good (for a more in-depth critique see Greenhalgh[29]). In reality, most people's experiences of scaling up is of a messy process of small wins, compromises, disappointments, and deadlocks that do not always lead to the result originally intended.

2.2 Ongoing Debates and Evolving Consensus

A number of debates recur in academic and applied efforts to achieve spread, scale-up, and sustainability in healthcare improvement.

2.2.1 Spread, Scale-Up, and Sustainability – in Sequence or in Parallel?

Spread, scale-up, and sustainability are sometimes depicted as three distinct and sequential phases in a linear improvement process. Spread is presented as taking place first when there is interest to adopt improvements beyond their original setting. Scale-up follows as it becomes clear what infrastructure will be needed in other settings for spread to be successful. Sustainability only receives attention after the first two processes are deemed complete during the initial (often poorly defined) implementation period.

However, as our overview of definitions in Section 2.1 suggests, it is more helpful to view spread, scale-up, and sustainability as inherently overlapping and interdependent processes.[26] For example, when an improvement effort achieves spread across an organisation or within the health service, it may be more likely to be sustained locally. Scale-up helps to ensure that the necessary infrastructure to support spread becomes available, while also increasing the chances of sustainability. A non-linear perspective recognises that spread, scale-up, and sustainability need to be pursued concurrently to be able to deal with the complexity of improvement efforts in contemporary health systems. Section 4 sets out two contrasting cases illustrating these points. NHS Scotland's video consulting service provides an additional example of spread being enabled by the early development of relevant infrastructure (e.g. technical equipment, organisational resources) and by considering sustainability from the outset.[31,32]

Rather than viewing spread, scale-up, and sustainability processes in mechanistic terms, we need to apply methods suitable for understanding complex adaptive systems that don't operate in a predictable and planned manner.[17,20,33,34] Viewing these translational processes as non-linear and mutually reinforcing also points to a different way of understanding improvement efforts and interventions – that is, as programmes formed by and interdependent with the context they are trying to influence, rather than something independent and optimised prior to widespread implementation. In short, we need to consider how to grow improvement efforts organically within the contexts of their implementation rather than try to build them mechanistically regardless of context. Organic growth perspectives are more attuned to local contexts and circumstances in all their social, cultural, and organisational complexity: they allow for local adaptation, contingency, negotiation, and dialogue, instead of rule-driven inflexible approaches and rigid patterns.

2.2.2 How to Balance Fidelity and Adaptability?

The academic literature features ongoing debate about the extent to which improvement interventions and their implementation strategies should adapt to local contexts and evolve over time.[35] Few studies describe how improvement programmes evolve and how implementation strategies are adapted to work at scale.[13,28] The terms implementation 'fidelity' or 'integrity' denote the extent to which an intervention or programme has been delivered as intended and in a more or less uniform way across all sites involved; the assumption is that high fidelity is more likely to lead to improvement.[36] Various ways of measuring and tracking fidelity have been devised (e.g. see the conceptual framework for implementation fidelity[36]), and checklists have been recommended to improve the description and replicability of interventions (e.g. see the TIDieR checklist[37]).

If unwarranted variations of process exist between different settings, this does impose learning overheads and creates risks at the system level.[38] However, there are tensions between standardisation and flexibility: How can spread and scale-up succeed if adaptation to local structures and a sense of local ownership are not encouraged?[39] But then, as Scheirer asks: 'If the adaptation of components is viewed as desirable at the local level, at what point is it no longer the "same" program?'[26] Are there essential components of a programme that need to be maintained and others that can be modified in different settings?

Some authors distinguish between the 'hard core' of an intervention (the features of an intervention that are deemed to be critical in leading to desired outcomes) and its 'soft periphery' (the wrap-around features that can and should be adapted to context).[14,40] For example, Denis et al. suggest that when introducing a new pharmaceutical treatment, the new drug formulation constitutes the hard core of the intervention, and the soft periphery refers to the organisational arrangements that enable changes to patient monitoring and follow-up, including decisions on who should be treated.[40] Yet, depending on the type of intervention, distinguishing between hard and soft components may be challenging, and what constitutes an irreducible feature in one context may need to become an adaptable feature in another.

Other authors suggest that instead of attempting to reproduce an intervention (or its implementation strategy) in the same *format* across settings, the emphasis should be on achieving the same *function*.[41] This focuses attention on understanding the *principles* by which an intervention is expected to generate change in one or more contexts (rather than its components or ingredients) – for example, through more informed use of programme theory.[9,41,42] Hawe et al. discuss the contrasting ways in which the same principle (e.g. educating patients about depression) can be standardised by format (e.g. all implementation sites need to distribute the same information leaflet for patients) or by function (e.g. sites need to develop their own ways of devising tailored information materials based on local population characteristics).[43] When it comes to spread, scale-up, and sustainability in complex systems, local adaptations and pragmatic adjustments become important to better adapt to local needs and continue meeting the intended function of improvement interventions over time (e.g. see Horton et al.[44] for survey evidence on how frequently adopters have to adapt interventions to context).

2.2.3 Sustainability of What?

Sustainability is an inherently ambiguous term since it embodies a tension between, on the one hand, an improvement intervention enduring in its current form (and hence potentially becoming obsolete over time as organisations adapt to accommodate it while perhaps overlooking new products and practices emerging elsewhere) and, on the other, the intervention changing over time or even being replaced by something more fit for purpose (as the organisation responds to a changing context).[11] Whereas the literature tends to assume that it is the innovation itself that should be sustained, the term 'sustainability' may also be used to mean sustainability of the service or health system. Increasingly, the term is also used to refer to sustainability of the planet and hence to considerations of reducing waste and pollution and working towards a greener future. Moreover, sustainability and scale-up may not always be desirable; de-implementation or scaling back in the sense of actively stopping obsolete practices may become an equally valuable goal towards improved safety, quality, and efficiency.[16,45]

Views in the literature vary on which aspects of sustainability to assess and at which level, for example, programme or system level. Some have called for tighter definitions of sustainability to ensure that all studies are using the term in the same way.[13] But perhaps it is more important to clarify, for any particular study, how the term is being used. Many studies take a relatively narrow view of sustainability as related only to the continuation of programme activities,[28] with some authors questioning what proportion and intensity of activities would establish a programme as sustained (especially after withdrawal of specific implementation support and capacity).[26] Others extend sustainability to encompass continued provision of beneficial outcomes for clients or service users, maintaining community attention to the problem addressed by the programme (e.g. after those who originally led implementation have moved on), sustaining community-level partnerships and coalitions (e.g. in relation to public health), or replicating the programme in other sites.[26,46,47] Different stakeholders will have different priorities and approaches to measuring sustainability – for example, commissioners may focus on savings, patients may view sustainability as related to continuation through their own treatment pathway, and providers may prioritise feasibility within staffing capacity and resources.

Øvretveit distinguishes between sustainability of impacts, projects, methods, and the capacity to improve quality.[21] This distinction is echoed by Greenhalgh et al., who discuss sustainability of the original vision and of the capacity for quality improvement so as to be able to balance emergent tensions.[11] They suggest that models of sustainability may be:

- 'intervention-focused (What if anything has been sustained?)'. Here, the focus is on the original programme and its components (studied using theoretical concepts such as fidelity and a more or less conventional logic model); or
- 'system-dynamic (How and why did change unfold as it did?)'. Here, the focus is on the innovation and its interacting and evolving context, including the interdependencies and uncertainties in a complex system (studied using mixed methods oriented to producing a rich and meaningful case study narrative).[11]

Greenhalgh et al. make the point that these seemingly incommensurable approaches may be fruitfully combined to depict how an innovation has *to some extent* been sustained as planned but has also *changed for good reason* to adapt to a changing context. Whereas basic logic-model evaluation of sustainability may involve a relatively simple check of whether original aims have been achieved, case studies of system-dynamic sustainability consider how both the innovation and the organisation have adapted dynamically, including an analysis of both intended and unintended consequences (which may be valued differently by different stakeholders).

2.2.4 What Are the Time Frames for Sustainability?

Beyond asking *what* counts as sustained improvement, it is also important to understand *when* an improvement might count as having been sustained. Research studies vary in the time frames they use to assess sustainability, but commonly limit measurement of outcomes to one or two years after implementation, depending on the type of intervention.[13,26] Funding may dictate how long it is possible for researchers to measure sustainability, as many healthcare improvement projects are carried out through time-limited, external collaborations. Healthcare organisations often have little internal capacity to continue measuring improvement sustainability (quantitatively and qualitatively) beyond standard performance targets mandated at system level.[13] So, to assess sustainability, a more strategic approach to medium-term and long-term measurement is needed, with appropriate justification for different types of interventions and adequate flexibility to capture changes over time. For example, Van de Ven describes how the Minnesota Innovation Research Programme coordinated longitudinal research across several innovation projects spanning almost two decades to develop process theory (i.e. explanations for how innovation unfolds over time). This was enabled by combining research grants and financial support from a range of sources (e.g. see Van de Ven and Poole[48] and Van de Ven[49]).

2.3 Influences on Spread, Scale-Up, and Sustainability

The literature provides evidence of extensive efforts to identify and understand what influences spread, scale-up, and sustainability. But although lists of (what are commonly framed as) 'barriers and facilitators' can be useful for considering some of the challenges that apply *across* improvement contexts, such lists rarely specify how challenges may play out in specific contexts and circumstances. Indeed, a limitation of the literature on barriers and facilitators is that they are usually depicted as fixed categories, whereas in reality different influences play out differently in different contexts. Something that acts as a barrier to change (e.g. regulation, public consultation, media coverage) in one study may prove to be a facilitator in another.[50]

Key contributors to successful change include the perceived value and feasibility of the improvement intervention – for example, the extent to which people being asked to adopt the change see it as adding value to their work (which may be different for different people) and as feasible to implement and sustain for the period required.[23,27] Demonstrating value may be easier in small-scale, localised improvement efforts, but when spread reaches across the health system the benefits of improvement efforts are more likely to become contested (e.g. as the way value is attributed will differ).[17] Other success factors include:

- intervention adaptability (i.e. its ability to meet the different objectives of potential adopters) depending on its level of maturity
- whether programme champions are involved as part of wider teams or structures promoting change, or only as lone enthusiasts

- the extent to which improvement efforts align with organisational priorities and routines, including broader interorganisational and community demand for improvement.[22,26]

Côté-Boileau et al.[23] provide a comprehensive synthesis of the 'complex web' of enabling conditions for spread, scale-up, and sustainability. These conditions include whether a programme can be adapted over time, whether leadership is distributed, and whether the pace of change is iterative (see Table 1 for a full list). Spread and scale-up efforts also need to consider potentially competing improvement interventions in specific organisational contexts and the highly political nature of healthcare organisations.[51] Consideration should also be given to the role of policy cycles, financial incentives, and other resources that can create organisational capacity for spread and scale-up efforts, as these are often overlooked.

Although Table 1 covers intraorganisational influences on spread, scale-up, and sustainability, it does not extend to interorganisational influences or features of the external context that may influence system-level spread and scale-up. Interorganisational networks influence spread as organisations compare their performance with each other and develop shared values around worthwhile improvement efforts that will help deliver their goals, especially in integrated systems such as the NHS. This occurs through informal networking between organisations but also through more formal networking opportunities, such as Beacon schemes and quality improvement collaboratives (see also the Element on collaboration-based approaches[52]).[14,53,54] Professional networks can act as additional levers for innovation spread given the strength of professional identities and communities in healthcare. Major improvement initiatives are also embedded in national policy programmes which influence their longevity and scale – for example, by providing dedicated funding or a political imperative for

Table 1 Enabling and limiting conditions for spread, scale-up, and sustainability

	Enabling conditions	**Limiting conditions**
Improvement or innovation	Adaptable	Static
Leadership	Distributed	Hierarchical
Accountability	Reciprocal	Unilateral
Context	Receptive	Tense
Timing and pace of change	Iterative	Linear
Management support	Empowering	Symbolic
Governance	Decentralised	Centralised

Adapted from Côté-Boileau et al.[23]

change (although the latter does not always strengthen internal organisational capacity for improvement overall, as it often requires diverting resources from other parts of the system).[14]

3 Approaches to Spread, Scale-Up, and Sustainability

3.1 Overview of Frameworks, Models, and Theories

Several frameworks, models, and theories have been proposed to explain and support spread, scale-up, and sustainability.[13,19,23,55] These include the Institute for Healthcare Improvement's Framework for Spread,[56] the NHS Sustainability Model,[27] Slaghuis et al.'s routinisation and institutionalisation instrument,[57] and the Dynamic Sustainability Framework.[15] Table 2 presents an overview of relevant frameworks, including their key focus and examples of clinical areas or settings where each approach has been used previously. Despite the abundance of frameworks, models, and theories, most have been used primarily in research rather than as applied tools for spread and scale-up.[13] When using research frameworks for applied purposes, part of the challenge is avoiding oversimplified or reductionist approaches.

Some spread, scale-up, and sustainability tools (derived from disciplines such as engineering and operations research) offer structured methods that aim to control predefined variables (e.g. organisational culture, staff attitudes) and assess the extent to which those variables affect the change process, both individually and collectively. Other types of structured models conceptualise the change effort as a clear sequence of steps (such as set-up, small-scale test-of-concept, further testing in different environments, and widespread scale-up) leading to spread, scale-up, and sustainability.[24] Sequential approaches make it easy to communicate what the process entails, but they can be misleading in that they create an impression that certain steps can only be taken in order of priority (in the aforementioned sequence, for example, that testing in multiple contrasting environments must not commence until a single, small-scale test of concept has been completed).

In contrast to structured and sequential tools, systems approaches (derived from complexity theory or the social sciences) foreground ecological factors and unpredictability and acknowledge that both the improvement intervention and the context(s) for its implementation context are evolving. Systems approaches question the value of quantifying particular determinants of spread, scale-up, and sustainability because different influences will play out very differently depending on circumstances. A crucial concept in a systems approach is path-dependency: the notion that, in any locality, there will be historical relationships, actions, and events that powerfully affect or set the

Table 2 Frameworks, models, and theories to explain and support spread, scale-up, and sustainability

	Focus and key components	Examples of clinical areas/settings where the framework has been applied
Dynamic Sustainability Framework[15]	Proposes that sustainability efforts focus on continuously optimising how the evolving intervention fits with the immediate implementation context, as well as with the broader system over time.	Cancer survivorship,[58] chronic care management, clinical guidelines, and psychotherapy.[15]
Institute for Healthcare Improvement's Framework for Going to Full Scale[24]	Describes a sequence of activities (set-up, developing a 'scalable unit', testing scale-up, going to full scale) needed for scale-up, alongside intervention adoption mechanisms (e.g. leadership) and support systems (e.g. technical infrastructure).	Care improvement programmes in Africa,[24] virtual care in Canada.[59]
Institute for Healthcare Improvement's Framework for Spread[56]	Focuses on six components that contribute to successful spread: leadership; relative advantage of the intervention; appropriate communication	Patient access in the US Veterans Health Administration, trauma-informed approach in paediatric care.[60]

Table 2 (cont.)

	Focus and key components	Examples of clinical areas/settings where the framework has been applied
	avenues; a strong social system for adoption; use of data to guide spread; and feedback to adapt the spread effort.	
NASSS (non-adoption, abandonment, and challenges to scale-up, spread, and sustainability) framework[8]	Emphasises multiple interacting influences across seven domains: the nature of the patient's illness or condition; type of technology or innovation; the value proposition; role of the adopter system; the organisation(s); the wider (including societal) context; and change over time.	Introduction of technological and service innovations in health and care.[61,62]
NHS Sustainability Model[27]	Accompanied by a practical guide, used as a diagnostic tool to identify implementation strengths and weaknesses and to predict the likelihood of improvement sustainability.	Quality improvement in the English NHS, whole systems collaborative for acute frailty.[63,64]
Normalisation process theory[65]	Explains the mechanisms by which new practices get introduced and	Several applications including telemedicine, telecare, and other

Table 2 (cont.)

	Focus and key components	Examples of clinical areas/settings where the framework has been applied
	become embedded in complex health and care settings.	improvement interventions in clinical care.[66,67]
Routinisation and institutionalisation instrument[57]	A quantitative instrument that measures quality improvement sustainability.	Quality improvement in chronic care,[68] emergency care.[69]
World Health Organization / ExpandNet[7]	An applied framework that guides strategic thinking on five interacting elements: the innovation, the user organisation, the environment, the resource team or organisation, and the scale-up strategy.	Global health and public health programmes.[70]
3S infrastructure approach[16]	Focuses on the role of context as an active agent in the change process, along with three other necessary components: human resources (people and groups at different management levels, with effective accountability, reporting and review processes); a strategy of actions and tasks; and monitoring and support systems.	Care transitions across large health systems in the USA.[16]

Table 2 (cont.)

	Focus and key components	Examples of clinical areas/settings where the framework has been applied
Multi-level perspective on sociotechnical transitions[71]	Theoretical approach that explains patterns of dynamic interactions between social and technical aspects of large-scale, complex innovation systems. Emphasises the roles and perspectives of end users and interest groups.	Environmental sustainability,[72] infrastructural programmes in science and technology, and healthcare innovation.[73]

scene for how a particular innovation or improvement effort is received. Path-dependencies may be geographical, legal, technological, sociocultural, commercial, or professional – or even a combination of all these. For example, contracts may have been signed with particular suppliers, the broadband service may require upgrading before a technological innovation can be supported, a recent failed project may have exhausted the goodwill and enthusiasm of staff, or there may be long-standing interpersonal rivalries between powerful individuals.

Although there are no firm rules to guide the choice of framework(s) in spread, scale-up, and sustainability efforts, familiarity with the different approaches will enable a more informed decision about which framework or tool is likely to best meet the needs and objectives of a change effort. As we have seen, systems approaches are more appropriate when the change effort is complex and likely to encounter multiple interdependencies. Apart from the routinisation and institutionalisation instrument, the majority of frameworks in Table 2 adopt a systems approach to some extent. Frameworks such as the NHS Sustainability Model and the World Health Organization and ExpandNet model for scaling up health service innovations have a more applied focus, while the NASSS framework, Dynamic Sustainability Framework, and 3S infrastructure approach have a dual research and applied purpose (the latter three are discussed in detail in Section 3.3).

3.2 Assumptions Underpinning Spread, Scale-Up, and Sustainability Approaches

Section 3.1 provides an overview of different frameworks, models, and theories on spread, scale-up, and sustainability. Those frameworks come from different disciplinary backgrounds, address different audiences, and embody different assumptions about the ways in which spread, scale-up, and sustainability are expected to happen. Some frameworks can be used to support a mechanistic approach to change, such as the systematic, planned application of structured improvement techniques and predetermined variables. Others emphasise that change is more complex, as the system in which an intervention is introduced tends to work in unpredictable, emergent ways and through interdependencies with other systems that cannot always be identified a priori. And some incorporate a social science orientation that focuses attention on the human and material influences in large-scale change efforts.[17] Table 3 sets out the key characteristics of mechanistic, complexity-informed, and social science-driven approaches to spread, scale-up, and sustainability.

Healthcare improvement efforts may draw on one or more of these approaches: they might focus primarily on a mechanistic approach because it provides more structure and certainty; or they may lean towards complexity and social science-oriented approaches in order to account for and manage unpredictability. Different members of an improvement team may contribute different ways of thinking. But when it comes to large-scale change efforts, which are likely to be contested (i.e. resisted), it may be important to use these three approaches in combination.[17] Many successful spread and scale-up programmes draw predominantly on one approach but also include elements of the other two.[17] Using elements from all three may help to achieve an appropriate balance between answering the (intervention-focused) question 'To what extent was the intervention spread or sustained as planned?' and developing a broader (system-focused) narrative around 'What changed and why?'[11]

3.3 Selected Frameworks

To better illustrate how spread, scale-up, and sustainability frameworks may contribute to healthcare improvement, we discuss three of them in more detail:

- Dynamic Sustainability Framework[15]
- 3S scale-up infrastructure approach[16]
- NASSS framework.[8]

Table 3 Three approaches to spread, scale-up, and sustainability

	Mechanistic approach	Complexity-informed approach	Social science-driven approach
Main focus	Evidence-based interventions.	The evolving and emergent properties of systems.	Social study of individuals, groups, organisations, and material practices.
Contribution	Provides a concrete, planned approach to the delivery and study of spread and scale-up.	Ecological view that emphasises the system's inherent unpredictability and need for adaptive change at multiple, interacting levels.	Foregrounds patterns of social behaviour and interaction, professional beliefs and values, and organisational routines and structures.
Key mechanisms of spread and scale-up	Uncertainty reduction, emphasis on fidelity and contextual influences.	Emergent properties of an interacting system – self organisation, management of interdependencies, and sense-making.	Social, professional, and organisational influences that shape (and are shaped by) individual and collective action.
Preferred methods for achieving spread and scale-up	Use structured, programmatic approaches to develop and replicate a complex intervention across multiple settings.	Gain a rich understanding of the case in its historical, sociopolitical, and organisational context. Use multiple methods flexibly and adaptively. Expect surprises and handle them creatively. Develop individuals and	Develop and apply theories of how individuals' behaviour and actions are influenced by interpersonal, material, organisational, professional, and other factors.

Table 3 (cont.)

	Mechanistic approach	Complexity-informed approach	Social science-driven approach
		organisations to be creative and resilient.	
Preferred methods for researching spread and scale-up	Metrics for measuring improvement (quantitatively) and systematic approach to exploring processes and mechanisms (qualitatively).	Case study approach using multiple qualitative and quantitative methods. Narrative can be used as a synthesising tool to capture complex chains of causation.	Ethnography, interview-based methods, and case narratives to provide insights into social interactions and contexts.
How success is measured	Replication of a particular service model or approach in multiple contexts ('fidelity').	Nuanced narrative about what changed and why, including (where relevant) how the intervention was adapted or why it was abandoned.	Theoretically informed and empirically justified explanations about human and organisational behaviour.

Adapted from Greenhalgh and Papoutsi[17]

We have chosen these frameworks because they foreground (to different degrees) spread, scale-up, and sustainability as adaptive processes in complex, social systems that are characterised by uncertainty, unpredictability, and emergence. They provide tools to be used reflectively, rather than mechanistically, to help manage complexity in spread, scale-up, and sustainability efforts and work through emerging tensions. In essence, they emphasise complexity-informed and social science-driven approaches to change, as outlined in Table 3.

3.3.1 The Dynamic Sustainability Framework

Chambers et al.'s Dynamic Sustainability Framework aims to help overcome challenges in spreading interventions beyond experimental settings. The framework cautions against over-reliance on fidelity and protocols when it comes to the success and sustainment of complex improvement efforts. Instead, the authors emphasise ongoing adaptations of improvement interventions over time in their implementation contexts.[15]

The framework has three key components:

- Intervention: interventions are primarily seen as being characterised by distinct components (e.g. clinical guidelines) which are intended to be delivered by designated individuals (e.g. clinicians) through specific delivery platforms (e.g. face-to-face, telephone) to achieve specific (often patient-based) outcomes.
- Practice setting or implementation context: the clinical or community context in which implementation happens is largely characterised by its human resources, organisational and technical infrastructures, and approaches to organisational learning and supervision (the framework places significant emphasis on learning healthcare systems).
- Ecological system: the broader ecological system comprises other clinical settings (where the intervention is not being implemented), the legislative and regulatory environment, market forces, and population characteristics.[15]

None of the three components is deemed static; rather, they are continuously evolving and changing in relation to external influences and each other (see Figure 1). Constant alignment or dynamic fit is needed based on learning and experimentation over time (see Box 2 for key principles). Because the framework focuses primarily on particular single interventions, it is best used in an organic way by teams looking to implement a guideline or protocol, for example.

Chambers et al. provide illustrative examples of how the framework could be applied in the areas of chronic care management, clinical guidelines, and psychotherapy implementation.[15] Urquhart et al. have used the framework in

---

Box 2 KEY PRINCIPLES OF THE DYNAMIC SUSTAINABILITY FRAMEWORK[15]

- Interventions are better maintained if optimised in adaptive ways to 'fit' their context, rather than prior to implementation; this also prevents 'voltage drop' (i.e. where improvement benefits identified experimentally diminish in real settings).
- Optimising the intervention in its context also drives stakeholders' (including patients') ongoing involvement and learning in the improvement process; organisational learning needs to be valued in the implementation setting.
- Progress measures can be used to allow adaptation and learning through feedback.

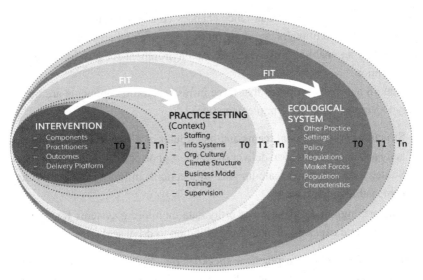

Figure 1 The Dynamic Sustainability Framework. The framework seeks to establish 'optimal' but dynamic 'fit' between the intervention, its implementation context and the broader system, in a balance that changes over time as each of the three components evolve (i.e. T0, T1, Tn). *Reproduced from Chambers et al.[15] in accordance with the terms of the Creative Commons Attribution Licence (http://creativecommons.org/licenses/by/4.0).*

their qualitative study of influences on the sustainability of innovations in cancer survivorship care.[58] Others have built on its principles to develop the foundations for their realist evaluation[74] and to extend research in cognitive work analysis.[75]

3.3.2 The 3S Scale-Up Infrastructure Approach

The crucial role of context, which is at the heart of the Dynamic Sustainability Framework, is also emphasised in Øvretveit et al.'s approach to developing a 3S (structure, strategy, supports) scale-up infrastructure.[16] Building on several years of research in this area,[76,77] the 3S approach distinguishes between the internal contexts (e.g. management support, leadership continuity) and external contexts (e.g. financing opportunities, favourable regulation) that influence improvement in practice. The authors argue that without a supportive organisational culture, strategic leadership, and accountability structures in place to drive improvement efforts, widespread change becomes difficult to achieve.[16] But instead of simply identifying contextual characteristics that may determine strong 'fit' with the intervention (as in the Dynamic Sustainability Framework), Øvretveit et al. encourage 'actions to increase readiness for change' and 'preparing contexts' so that the chances for successful scale-up are maximised.[16] Practitioners can draw on this approach when seeking to create and sustain an enabling infrastructure and environment for any improvement intervention.

The 3S approach proposes that three infrastructural components are necessary to support large-scale implementation:

- Structure: organisational teams and individuals at different levels with capacity and accountability to deliver scale-up, supported by a reporting process.
- Strategy: an organised scale-up plan with actions, milestones, and allocated responsible individuals.
- Support: high-quality and trustworthy data monitoring systems for periodic reviews, and expertise in adaptive facilitation to drive scale-up.

The approach includes a practical checklist for improvers to help guide 3S infrastructure development. The checklist provides a series of improvement-related questions about process for prioritisation, structure of accountability, flexibility for adaptation, and support available from leaders, facilitators, and researchers. It suggests asking informed observers to attribute scores of 0–5 for how much of each element is present in the development context. Low scores for some elements can suggest areas where attention is needed to improve the chances of success of the scale-up programme.[16]

Given its applied focus, there are few published examples of this approach, but those leading improvement efforts may find the explanation provided by Øvretveit et al. on care transitions across large health systems in the USA helpful.[16]

3.3.3 The NASSS Framework

Instead of treating improvement efforts as linear and simplistic, the NASSS framework aims to understand and explain unpredictability, uncertainty, dynamic interactions, and interdependencies. Drawing on complexity theory and social science for its dominant underpinning theoretical lens, Greenhalgh and her team developed the framework in 2017 to address persistent problems related to technological but also other types of innovation projects in health and care.[8]

NASSS includes seven domains (with associated sub-domains) in which complexity manifests to varying degrees in technology projects (see Figure 2):

- the nature of the health condition or illness
- the type of technology (or intervention)

- the value proposition (both financial, e.g. return on investment, and non-financial, e.g. benefits to patients)
- the role of intended adopters
- organisational capacity and other support structures
- the complexity of the wider system
- the potential for continuous embedding and adaptation over time.

Each domain can be characterised as simple, complicated, or complex. For example, a simple illness or condition (e.g. a sprained ankle) has clear diagnostic criteria and its management can be predictable; a complicated illness (e.g. some types of cancer) may be more challenging to manage but would still follow a clinically predictable path; a complex illness (e.g. psychosis) is more likely to require ongoing care that takes into account comorbidities and other social factors.

Programmes where multiple domains are characterised as complicated (there are multiple interacting components or issues) may encounter more spread and scale-up challenges. Programmes where multiple domains are complex (dynamic, unpredictable, not easily disaggregated into constituent components) will be less likely to become sustained without significant effort.[61] What matters is not just complexity within the domains themselves, but also the interactions and inter-dependencies between the domains over time, as the arrows in Figure 2 illustrate.

The NASSS framework aims to:

- inform the design of technology
- support planning for implementation, spread, or scale-up
- contribute to early identification of innovations where increased complexity is likely to limit success
- increase learning by explaining programme failures.

The framework is not intended as a checklist, but as a sensitising device to facilitate construction of a rich narrative synthesising different perspectives in unfolding technology programmes. Several researchers and policymakers have used the NASSS framework to understand, plan, and explain the journeys of technology projects, including video consultations, remote monitoring, and decision support (e.g. see Abimbola et al.[79]). A series of practical tools for improvement teams based on NASSS is described in Box 3.

4 Spread, Scale-Up, and Sustainability in Action

In this section, we present two case narratives that describe spread and scale-up efforts in two healthcare improvement programmes. We provide a brief background for each programme before discussing the influences that led to their partial successes and failures.

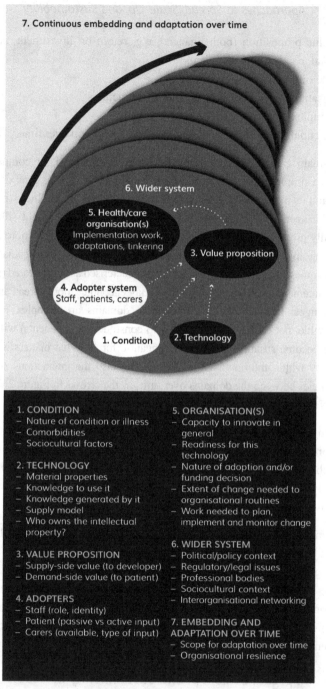

Figure 2 The NASSS framework for studying non-adoption, abandonment, and challenges to spread, scale-up, and sustainability of technology projects in health and care organisations

> **Box 3 NASSS-CAT: A PRACTICAL TOOLKIT**
>
> Through a process of co-design, the NASSS framework has been combined with a validated complexity assessment tool (CAT) to produce a practical toolkit (NASSS-CAT) supporting teams to deliver spread, scale-up, and sustainability in healthcare technology projects. NASSS-CAT provides ways of breaking down and discussing complexity so that teams can plan their improvement projects and address ongoing challenges in a participatory way. The toolkit[80] can be accessed in different formats (Word, Google Sheets, Excel, Office 365).

4.1 Spread and Scale-Up of an Obstetric Emergency Training Package

4.1.1 How Was the Intervention Developed, Spread, and Scaled Up?

PRactical Obstetric Multi-Professional Training (PROMPT) is a multi-professional training package for obstetric emergencies in maternity units. Based on a local course that was originally developed in 2000 to address local training needs at Southmead Hospital in Bristol, the training package aims to help midwives, obstetricians, anaesthetists, and other members of multi-professional maternity teams deliver safe and effective maternity care.[62,81]

Following early evidence of organisational and system-level benefits from delivery of the training package in both real-world and simulation settings,[82,83] a clinical effectiveness study identified improvements in staff knowledge, teamwork, and outcomes for mothers and babies.[84–87] In 2008, the Bristol team developed a 'train the trainer' (T3) model for PROMPT, whereby a multi-professional team attend training and learn how to deliver courses in their own maternity unit. Key to this training model was the 'course in a box' concept. It sought to ensure that after being trained themselves, the maternity unit teams are provided with wide-ranging training resources (course and trainers' manuals, scenarios, videos, clinical algorithms, and emergency boxes) that they can adapt and use to deliver training at local sites. Initial course materials were published with the support of the Royal College of Obstetricians and Gynaecologists,[83] until the PROMPT Maternity Foundation (a registered charity in England and Wales) was set up in 2012. Second and third editions of the 'course in a box' were published in 2012 (PROMPT 2) and 2017 (PROMPT 3), and its continued local use has been associated with sustained improvements in outcomes.[88]

In 2014, the PROMPT Maternity Foundation ran a stepped-wedge rollout of PROMPT across 12 maternity units in Scotland (the THISTLE Study).[89] And in 2017, Welsh Risk Pool funded the rollout and evaluation of PROMPT in 12 maternity units in Wales (PROMPT Wales).[90] In 2018, the PROMPT Maternity Foundation was awarded funding to work with a social franchising team, Spring Impact, to understand how to sustain PROMPT use and best practices at local level. An enhanced implementation support package, the PROMPT Partnership Programme, was developed in 2018 and piloted at five sites in the UK.[87] Evaluation of this enhanced support package demonstrated that scaling up was possible and learnings from the programme have been included in the fourth PROMPT training package, the PROMPT Annual Update.

Most maternity units across the UK have either attended a PROMPT T3 programme or downloaded the more recent PROMPT digital training resources and integrated implementation programme. Based on data held by the PROMPT Maternity Foundation, the PROMPT Annual Update package has been accessed by 104 maternity units across the UK as of May 2023. In addition, PROMPT has also been introduced (in its original or adapted format) in 15 countries around the world, and a further 10 countries have sent maternity teams to receive training, although the actual scale of local implementation is not actively monitored (data until May 2023).

4.1.2 What Influenced Spread and Scale-Up?

Achieving this degree of scale-up and spread took many years with diverse influences from multiple contributors. In the UK, pump-prime funding from the Royal College of Obstetricians and Gynaecologists was important for initial rollout.[83] There has been a plethora of published evidence describing the positive impacts of PROMPT training on safety and effectiveness of maternity care and this has justified both initial uptake and later spread, nationally and internationally, by providing a compelling value proposition for adoption.[83]

Spread and scale-up were also strongly influenced by the external landscape, in particular the policy environment. For example, NHS Resolution had recommended local multi-professional training for those delivering maternity care. The Clinical Negligence Scheme for Trusts Maternity Incentive Scheme in England and, in Australia, the Victorian Managed Insurance Authority incentivise providers to meet safety actions to improve maternity care.[83] This type of policy and regulatory infrastructure has been key for sustainability to date.

Those behind the development of PROMPT also played a key role in encouraging demand and facilitating spread, both through their own leadership and by identifying local champions for adoption in maternity units.[83] This core, multi-professional PROMPT team of clinicians helped build supportive relationships and networks for spread, for example by talking about PROMPT training at professional events and within formal and informal networks. This helped to raise awareness and stimulate interest and demand. The team behind the intervention also worked with academics to understand the social and relational nature of interventions and how this can impact on successful implementation and spread. Although initial spread was mainly organic and not grounded in an explicit strategy, understanding social and relational influences helped codify success factors and informed approaches to spread later on.[83]

Various features of the intervention itself have also supported spread and sustainability at some sites. They include the user-friendly, localised training model, meaning that healthcare staff are not required to travel to simulation centres, more staff from a single unit can benefit at the same time, and locally delivered training is more cost-effective than training in a simulation centre.[83] A train the trainer model also supports both spread and sustainability as the training effort is not dependent on external trainers and the course materials can be adapted to support local implementation.[83] And the option of external implementation support (part of the PROMPT Partnership Programme) can help sites which might otherwise struggle to deliver and sustain the training fully autonomously and over time – for example, because of difficulty in securing management buy-in and commitment to release staff time to attend training, or delays in implementation of local training following initial attendance at the PROMPT train the trainer session.[87]

The PROMPT core team have identified some key influences that are important in ensuring future sustainability, including:

- sustaining policy-level support
- being able to nurture communities of practice around the training package
- ensuring implementation fidelity of core components (while recognising the importance of adaptability to a local context as well)
- nurturing receptive organisational environments, including organisational support for staff to attend and deliver training
- conducive team relationships in the settings that are implementing the improvement effort
- local champions
- ongoing trouble-shooting support from the PROMPT Maternity Foundation.[83]

4.2 Spread and Scale-Up of a Patient Safety Checklist

4.2.1 How Was the Intervention Developed, Spread, and Scaled Up?

Older patients may suffer disproportionate levels of harm due to inconsistent implementation of accepted clinical standards in non-specialist settings.[91] The Frailsafe collaborative sought to address this challenge by spreading implementation of a patient safety checklist in 12 acute hospitals across the UK. The idea behind the checklist was to ensure that a number of evidence-based interventions were completed as soon as possible after admission. The checklist, which was refined and eventually standardised during the programme, consisted of two parts: a screening phase to identify older patients in need of specialist assessment; and confirmation (where appropriate) that key assessments (e.g. dementia, delirium, mobility, among others) had been completed.[91]

Checklist use was expected to result in more reliable clinical assessment to prevent harm, in improved communication between clinical teams (especially frailty and acute care teams), and in less hierarchical ways of working. Clinical staff were encouraged to use the checklist to 'challenge' each other around appropriate and timely completion of assessments.[91] The spread and scale-up effort was supported by the Frailsafe collaborative (based on the Breakthrough Series model[92]), which brought together the 12 hospital teams alongside a team of geriatricians and quality improvement experts.[91] The project was also supported by a professional organisation for geriatricians in the UK and received significant attention at the time.

4.2.2 What Influenced Spread and Scale-Up?

Despite the initiative's highly structured quality improvement approach and enthusiasm among participating sites, a mixed-methods evaluation across the 12 UK sites identified challenges in spreading and scaling up use of the checklist within (and beyond) the collaborative.[93] Hospital teams did perceive value in adopting a quick shorthand approach to identifying older people in need of additional assessment, and they found the checklist useful for highlighting gaps in the ways assessments were carried out locally. However, they also recognised that the checklist's contribution to patient safety was limited because completion of assessments did not always lead to better patient care. And even when use of the checklist identified that an assessment had not been done, this did not always lead to further action. Use of the checklist was often at odds with the reality of admission routines and already established, culturally complex ways of working and communicating in different clinical settings.[93]

To our knowledge, checklist adoption remained limited to improvement teams participating in the Frailsafe collaborative and rarely extended to other hospital teams. Its introduction was not sufficient to broker new ways of working across geriatric medicine and acute care, nor to change communication patterns in hierarchical multidisciplinary teams. In contrast to the original programme design, the checklist was often completed by clinicians independently rather than in the context of a clinical discussion with other team members, or it was used by senior doctors to check whether more junior members of staff had completed their duties. Such dynamics were more visible in clinical settings where isolated working and strong hierarchies were prevalent. The checklist appeared to be used more meaningfully by teams that already had well-developed and positive collaboration styles. Although leadership at programme level was strong, the extent to which local champions were able to promote change in their settings and to garner organisational support varied.[93]

Spread and scale-up were limited because they were perceived as primarily technical and mechanistic processes; less attention was paid to the practical everyday accomplishment of clinical work in different settings, to established routines and interprofessional dynamics, norms, and values, and to dynamically changing local organisational contexts. Adapting the patient safety intervention locally to respond to specific needs and align with pre-existing processes might have enabled further spread. Identifying ways to link with accountability structures, support established teamwork patterns and relationships, as well as involve other stakeholders, such as patients and carers, could also have supported more widespread adoption.[93]

5 Critical Reflections and Implications for Improvement Research and Practice

Widespread and sustained uptake of improvement interventions (already successful in the context of origin) has potential to increase efficiency, quality, and safety in healthcare. But while well-defined interventions with concrete evidence of positive impact may be easier to replicate (e.g. as in some aspects of the PROMPT training programme presented in Section 4), major system-level interventions, such as the introduction of new ways of remote consulting, may prove difficult to spread and sustain (see also Greenhalgh et al.[61]). In this Element, we argue for more attention to complexity and social influences to better support large-scale change, rather than treating interventions as standardisable, self-contained packages that can be mechanically transferred across settings.

Instead of trying to solve abstracted or oversimplified versions of improvement problems, we need to focus efforts on increasing capacity for improvement and on addressing inherent tensions in the improvement process. The following principles – focused on the role of those leading improvement and intervention 'users' (direct or indirect) – may help to improve spread and scale-up:[17]

- Develop adaptive capability in staff – so that they can make good judgements with limited data and self-organise to adapt interventions for intended aims.
- Give attention to human relationships – so that people can work together to embed improvements with reciprocity and goodwill, which are often needed in complex projects.
- Productively harness conflict – because complex problems give rise to contesting views which need to be voiced and brought together in a constructive way.

Spread and scale-up cannot always be neatly planned and executed. Therefore, sense-making (i.e. 'the process by which people, individually and collectively, assign meaning to experience and link it to action'[17]) and focused experimentation need to be encouraged. Those involved in implementation need to be recognised as autonomous, active partners in the change process (rather than as passive implementers of interventions designed elsewhere).[94] This means recognising the role of human actors, the professional values by which their work is organised, their established routines, and the tools at their disposal, in more or less formalised organisational contexts.[51] What counts as a credible source of improvement data will vary between professional communities, as will 'the nature of quality, accuracy or data relevance concerns that need to be borne in mind'.[95]

Co-designing with intended users (either directly or indirectly affected by the intervention) could lead to better adaptations of interventions in systems-focused ways that take account of healthcare staff as professionals driven by values and norms, and patients as partners actively engaged in shaping the service and the improvement effort (see also the Element on co-producing and co-designing[96]).[31] It is important to foster ongoing collaborations between communities, policymakers, and implementation teams, to be able to advance translation in practice.[97]

A number of practical guides are available to support those leading improvement (e.g. see Hemmings et al.[3] and Albury et al.[22]). They include guidance at the level of the improvement initiative, for example, around creating demand for improvement and finding a balance between fidelity, adaptability, and quality. Significant scope remains for more effective use of spread, scale-up, and sustainability frameworks and assessment tools in practice (such as the ones presented in this Element). Better use of theoretical frameworks would support transferability of learning across settings but also allow for detailed evaluation to surface how unique aspects of different programmes become co-shaped in implementation settings across health systems. Attention is also needed to instances where spread and sustainability are not always desirable, for example, if the evidence base for an intervention changes over time or if an intervention contradicts or confounds other important practices. A growing literature explores de-implementation and abandonment of interventions, including strategies for restricting or reducing interventions when no longer delivering the outcomes intended.[45]

Supporting spread also has implications for the wider improvement and innovation ecosystem. For example, it is important that policymakers provide sufficient financial support to enable innovations to achieve sustainable spread and wide-scale impact within an appropriate time frame. However, this should not be at the expense of smaller, localised interventions for which spread and scale may not be possible but which nevertheless have a significant impact on a local need or population. Policymakers should strive to achieve an effective balance between the two.[22]

Beyond funding, many other system-level actions can play a role. They include behavioural and cultural levers, in addition to financial and structural interventions (e.g. see Horton et al.[44]). Attention is needed to the types of incentives and accountabilities likely to support spread and sustainability of proven good practices (e.g. embedding accountability as part of inspection regimes, in a way attuned to local needs).[73] Policy actions also have a role to play in nurturing the skills and capabilities necessary for improvement, starting from an early stage (e.g. as part of medical education curricula) as well as through continuing professional development, including attention to social skills that can foster effective relationships and learning networks.

6 Conclusions

In their article on the scale-up of health innovations in low-income and middle-income countries, Spicer et al. argue that 'scaling-up is a craft not a science'.[98] In this final section, we summarise key learning for those who engage in and study this craft.

From a practice perspective, improvement efforts would benefit from considering the potential for spread, scale-up, and sustainability early on, rather than as an afterthought. There is a need to move beyond a narrow focus on specific interventions to consider the system in which they will be embedded and the people who will be involved, directly or indirectly, in the improvement process. A commitment to adaptations that fulfil the same purpose in different settings, rather than interventions implemented rigidly without local tailoring, is likely to be valuable. Enabling conditions such as distributed leadership, adequate management support, and an environment receptive to improvement effort and iterative change all require constant cultivation and an organic growth mindset that prioritises negotiation, dialogue, and relationships rather than mechanistic approaches.

From a research perspective, there is a need for robust, longitudinal and mixed methods evaluations of spread, scale-up, and sustainability efforts, including ethnographic and narrative approaches that surface emergence and interdependencies. Currently emphasis is placed primarily on spread and scale-up of single improvement interventions, with little attention paid to organisational life playing out in the midst of several improvement initiatives occurring in parallel. Further research is needed to better understand spread and scale-up of combinatorial approaches (i.e. multiple competing or reinforcing initiatives), and to tease out interactions between improvement efforts, understand how to support improvers with managing multiple improvement opportunities, and consider how best to de-implement widespread routinised practices.

Complexity-informed and social science-oriented approaches can provide a useful lens to consider in research design and in equipping improvement practitioners with the language and tools to think about and operationalise spread, scale-up, and sustainability.

7 Further Reading

Further Information for Those Leading Improvement

- Hemmings et al.[3] – Nuffield Trust report synthesising learning on scale and spread for innovators and policymakers.
- Albury et al.[22] and Horton et al.[44] – reports by the Health Foundation (and the Innovation Unit) with practical examples on successful spread in healthcare.
- Maher et al.[27] and NHS Horizons[99] – resources on spread and adoption of improvements in the NHS (including the NHS Sustainability Model and guide).
- World Health Organization[7] and Institute for Healthcare Improvement[18] – guidance for scaling up innovations.

Review Papers and Books

- Côté-Boileau et al.[23] – summarise the literature on spread, scale-up, and sustainability.
- Braithwaite et al.[13] and Lennox et al.[55] – provide an overview of the literature on sustainability.

Rich Empirical Studies

- Øvretveit and Staines[76] – case study of the Jönköping quality programme.
- Dixon-Woods et al.[9] – ethnographic study of a patient safety programme (explaining why it failed to spread as expected).
- Greenhalgh et al.[11] – case study on sustainability of whole-system change.

Critical Discussion of Mainstream Approaches

- Hawe et al.[43] – argue for attention to the dynamic properties of context and complex ecological systems.
- Øvretveit[77] – describes three approaches to spreading improvement: hierarchical control, participatory adaptation, and facilitated evolution.
- Greenhalgh and Papoutsi[17] – suggest a shift from mechanistic approaches to spread and scale-up towards adopting complexity-informed and social science-oriented perspectives.

Contributors

Chrysanthi Papoutsi carried out the background literature review, and drafted and revised the Element. Sonja Marjanovic drafted the first case narrative following an interview with the programme designers. She also contributed to the writing and reviewed the Element. Trisha Greenhalgh contributed to the writing and reviewed the Element. All authors have approved the final version.

Conflicts of Interest

None.

Acknowledgements

We thank the peer reviewers for their insightful comments and recommendations to improve the Element. A list of peer reviewers is published at www.cambridge.org/IQ-peer-reviewers. We would also like to thank the PROMPT team for providing information on the development of their improvement programme.

Funding

This Element was funded by THIS Institute (The Healthcare Improvement Studies Institute, www.thisinstitute.cam.ac.uk). THIS Institute is strengthening the evidence base for improving the quality and safety of healthcare. THIS Institute is supported by a grant to the University of Cambridge from the Health Foundation – an independent charity committed to bringing about better health and healthcare for people in the UK.

About the Authors

Chrysanthi Papoutsi is an Associate Professor at the Nuffield Department of Primary Care Health Sciences. Her research interests include the interdisciplinary study of digital health and innovation, the complex reconfiguration of health services to support specific groups, and the use of technology and artificial intelligence to manage patient safety.

Trisha Greenhalgh is Professor of Primary Care at the Nuffield Department of Primary Care Health Sciences. Her research seeks to celebrate and retain the traditional and humanistic aspects of medicine while also embracing the unparalleled opportunities of contemporary science and technology to improve health outcomes and relieve suffering.

Sonja Marjanovic directs RAND Europe's portfolio of research in the field of healthcare innovation, industry, and policy. Her work provides decision-makers with evidence and insights to support innovation and improvement in healthcare systems, and to support the translation of innovation into societal benefits for healthcare services and population health.

Creative Commons License

References

1. NHS England. *NHS Long Term Plan*. London: NHS; 2019. www
   .longtermplan.nhs.uk (accessed 22 January 2023).
2. Marjanovic S, Altenhofer M, Hocking L, et al. *Innovating for Improved
   Healthcare: Policy and Practice for a Thriving NHS*. Santa Monica, CA:
   RAND Corporation, 2020. https://doi.org/10.7249/RR2711.
3. Hemmings N, Hutchings R, Castle-Clarke S, Palmer W. *Achieving Scale and
   Spread: Learning for Innovators and Policy-makers*. London: Nuffield
   Trust; 2020. www.nuffieldtrust.org.uk/research/achieving-scale-and-spread-
   learning-for-innovators-and-policy-makers (accessed 22 January 2023).
4. Agency for Healthcare Research and Quality. *Topic Collection: Taking
   Innovations to Scale*. Rockville, MD: AHRQ; 2021. https://innovations
   .ahrq.gov/topic-collections/taking-innovations-scale (accessed 22 January
   2023).
5. Milat AJ, Newson R, King L, et al. A guide to scaling up population health
   interventions. *Public Health Res Pract* 2016; 26(1): c2611604. https://doi
   .org/10.17061/phrp2611604.
6. Hanson K, Cleary S, Schneider H, Tantivess S, Gilson L. Scaling up health
   policies and services in low- and middle-income settings. *BMC Health Serv
   Res* 2010; 10(1): I1. https://doi.org/10.1186/1472-6963-10-S1-I1.
7. World Health Organization. *Practical Guidance for Scaling Up Health
   Service Innovations*. Geneva, Switzerland: WHO; 2009. https://apps
   .who.int/iris/handle/10665/44180 (accessed 22 January 2023).
8. Greenhalgh T, Wherton J, Papoutsi C, et al. Beyond adoption: A new
   framework for theorizing and evaluating nonadoption, abandonment, and
   challenges to the scale-up, spread, and sustainability of health and care
   technologies (NASSS framework). *J Med Internet Res* 2017; 19(11): e367.
   https://doi.org/10.2196/jmir.8775.
9. Dixon-Woods M, Leslie M, Tarrant C, Bion J. Explaining Matching
   Michigan: An ethnographic study of a patient safety program. *Implement
   Sci* 2013; 8: 70. https://doi.org/10.1186/1748-5908-8-70.
10. Greenhalgh T, Wherton J, Shaw S, et al. Infrastructure revisited: An
    ethnographic case study of how health information infrastructure shapes
    and constrains technological innovation. *J Med Internet Res* 2019; 21(12):
    e16093. https://doi.org/10.2196/16093.
11. Greenhalgh T, Macfarlane F, Barton-Sweeney C, Woodard F. 'If we build it,
    will it stay?' A case study of the sustainability of whole-system change in

London. *Milbank Q* 2012; 90: 516–47. https://doi.org/10.1111/j.1468-0009 .2012.00673.x.

12. James H, Papoutsi C, Wherton J, Greenhalgh T, Shaw S. Spread, scale-up, and sustainability of video consulting in health care: A systematic review and synthesis guided by the NASSS Framework. *J Med Internet Res* 2021; 23(1): e23775. https://doi.org/10.2196/23775.

13. Braithwaite J, Ludlow K, Testa L, et al. Built to last? The sustainability of healthcare system improvements, programmes and interventions: A systematic integrative review. *BMJ Open* 2020; 10: e036453. https://doi .org/10.1136/bmjopen-2019-036453.

14. Greenhalgh T, Robert G, Macfarlane F, Bate P, Kyriakidoy O. Diffusion of innovations in service organizations: Systematic review and recommendations. *Milbank Q* 2004; 82: 581–629. https://doi.org/10.1111/ j.0887-378X.2004.00325.x.

15. Chambers DA, Glasgow RE, Stange KC. The dynamic sustainability framework: Addressing the paradox of sustainment amid ongoing change. *Implement Sci* 2013; 8: 117. https://doi.org/10.1186/1748-5908-8-117.

16. Øvretveit J, Garofalo L, Mittman B. Scaling up improvements more quickly and effectively. *Int J Qual Health Care* 2017; 29: 1014–9. https:// doi.org/10.1093/intqhc/mzx147

17. Greenhalgh T, Papoutsi C. Spreading and scaling up innovation and improvement. *BMJ* 2019; 365: l2068. https://doi.org/10.1136/bmj.l2068.

18. Institute for Healthcare Improvement. *How-To Guide: Sustainability and Spread.* Cambridge, MA: IHI; 2008. www.ihi.org/resources/Pages/Tools/ HowtoGuideSustainabilitySpread.aspx (accessed 22 January 2023).

19. Lennox L, Maher L, Reed J. Navigating the sustainability landscape: A systematic review of sustainability approaches in healthcare. *Implement Sci* 2018; 13: 27. https://doi.org/10.1186/s13012-017-0707-4.

20. Norton WE, McCannon CJ, Schall MW, Mittman BS. A stakeholder-driven agenda for advancing the science and practice of scale-up and spread in health. *Implement Sci* 2012; 7: 118. https://doi.org/10.1186/1748-5908- 7-118.

21. Øvretveit J. Implementing, sustaining, and spreading quality improvement. In: The Joint Commission. *From Front Office to Front Line: Essential Issues for Health Care Leaders.* 2nd ed. Chicago, IL: The Joint Commission; 2011: 159–76. www.researchgate.net/publication/ 310480495_Implementing_sustaining_and_spreading_quality_improvem ent (accessed 22 January 2023).

22. Albury D, Beresford T, Dew S, et al. *Against the Odds: Successfully Scaling Innovation in the NHS.* London: Innovation Unit & The Health

Foundation; 2020. www.health.org.uk/publications/against-the-odds-successfully-scaling-innovation-in-the-nhs (accessed 22 January 2023).

23. Côté-Boileau É, Denis J-L, Callery B, Sabean M. The unpredictable journeys of spreading, sustaining and scaling healthcare innovations: A scoping review. *Health Res Policy Syst* 2019; 17: 84. https://doi.org/10.1186/s12961-019-0482-6.

24. Barker PM, Reid A, Schall MW. A framework for scaling up health interventions: Lessons from large-scale improvement initiatives in Africa. *Implement Sci* 2015; 11: 12. https://doi.org/10.1186/s13012-016-0374-x.

25. Cox A, Spiegelhalter K, Marangozov R, et al. *NHS Innovation Accelerator Evaluation: Final Report*. Brighton: Institute for Employment Studies; 2018. www.employment-studies.co.uk/resource/nhs-innovation-accelerator-evalu ation (accessed 22 January 2023).

26. Scheirer MA. Is sustainability possible? A review and commentary on empirical studies of program sustainability. *Am J Eval* 2005; 26: 320–47. https://doi.org/10.1177/1098214005278752.

27. Maher L, Gustafson D, Evans A. *Sustainability Model and Guide*. Coventry: Institute for Innovation and Improvement; 2010. www.eng land.nhs.uk/improvement-hub/publication/sustainability-model-and-guide (accessed 26 June 2023).

28. Moore JE, Mascarenhas A, Bain J, Straus SE. Developing a comprehensive definition of sustainability. *Implement Sci* 2017; 12: 110. https://doi.org/10 .1186/s13012-017-0637-1.

29. Greenhalgh T. *How To Spread Good Ideas*. London: National Co-ordinating Centre for NHS Service Delivery and Organisation; 2004. http://citeseerx.ist.psu.edu/viewdoc/download?doi=10.1.1.127.336 &rep=rep1&type=pdf (accessed 22 January 2023).

30. Proctor E, Luke D, Calhoun A, et al. Sustainability of evidence-based healthcare: Research agenda, methodological advances, and infrastructure support. *Implement Sci* 2015; 10: 88. https://doi.org/10.1186/s13012-015-0274-5.

31. Papoutsi C, Wherton J, Shaw S, Morrison C, Greenhalgh T. Putting the social back into sociotechnical: Case studies of co-design in digital health. *J Am Med Inform Assoc* 2021; 28: 284–93. https://doi.org/10.1093/jamia/ ocaa197.

32. Wherton J, Greenhalgh T. *Video Consulting Service Evaluation 2019–2020: Report*. Edinburgh: Scottish Government; 2020. www.gov.scot/publications/ evaluation-attend-anywhere-near-video-consulting-service-scotland-2019-20-main-report (accessed 22 January 2023).

33. Shaw J, Shaw S, Wherton J, Hughes G, Greenhalgh T. Studying scale-up and spread as social practice: Theoretical introduction and empirical case study. *J Med Internet Res* 2017; 19: e244. https://doi.org/10.2196/jmir.7482.

34. Greene MC, Huang TTK, Giusto A, et al. Leveraging systems science to promote the implementation and sustainability of mental health and psychosocial interventions in low- and middle-income countries. *Harv Rev Psychiatry* 2021; 29(4): 262–77. https://doi.org/10.1097/HRP.0000000000000306.

35. Slaughter SE, Hill JN, Snelgrove-Clarke E. What is the extent and quality of documentation and reporting of fidelity to implementation strategies: A scoping review. *Implement Sci* 2015; 10: 129. https://doi.org/10.1186/s13012-015-0320-3.

36. Carroll C, Patterson M, Wood S, et al. A conceptual framework for implementation fidelity. *Implement Sci* 2007; 2: 40. https://doi.org/10.1186/1748-5908-2-40.

37. Hoffmann TC, Glasziou PP, Boutron I, et al. Better reporting of interventions: Template for intervention description and replication (TIDieR) checklist and guide. *BMJ* 2014; 348: g1687. https://doi.org/10.1136/bmj.g1687.

38. Dixon-Woods M, Martin GP. Does quality improvement improve quality? *Future Hospital Journal* 2016; 3: 191–4. https://doi.org/10.7861/futurehosp.3-3-191.

39. Papoutsi C, Boaden R, Foy R, Grimshaw J, Rycroft-Malone J. Challenges for implementation science. In: Raine R, Fitzpatrick R, Barratt H, et al., editors. *Challenges, Solutions and Future Directions in the Evaluation of Service Innovations in Health Care and Public Health.* Southampton: NIHR Journals Library; 2016: 121–32. https://doi.org/10.3310/hsdr04160.

40. Denis J-L, Hébert Y, Langley A, Lozeau D, Trottier L-H. Explaining diffusion patterns for complex health care innovations. *Health Care Manage Rev* 2002; 27: 60–73. https://doi.org/10.1097/00004010-200207000-00007.

41. Hawe P, Shiell A, Riley T. Theorising interventions as events in systems. *Am J Community Psychol* 2009; 43: 267–76. https://doi.org/10.1007/s10464-009-9229-9.

42. Davidoff F, Dixon-Woods M, Leviton L, Michie S. Demystifying theory and its use in improvement. *BMJ Qual Saf* 2015; 24: 228–38. https://doi.org/10.1136/bmjqs-2014-003627.

43. Hawe P, Shiell A, Riley T. Complex interventions: how 'out of control' can a randomised controlled trial be? *BMJ* 2004; 328: 1561–3. https://doi.org/10.1136/bmj.328.7455.1561.

44. Horton T, Illingworth J, Warburton W. *The Spread Challenge*. London: The Health Foundation; 2018. www.health.org.uk/publications/the-spread-challenge (accessed 20 March 2022).

45. Norton WE, Chambers DA. Unpacking the complexities of de-implementing inappropriate health interventions. *Implement Sci* 2020; 15: 2. https://doi.org/10.1186/s13012-019-0960-9.

46. Shediac-Rizkallah MC, Bone LR. Planning for the sustainability of community-based health programs: Conceptual frameworks and future directions for research, practice and policy. *Health Educ Res* 1998; 13: 87–108. https://doi.org/10.1093/her/13.1.87.

47. Scheirer MA, Dearing JW. An agenda for research on the sustainability of public health programs. *Am J Public Health* 2011; 101: 2059–67. https://doi.org/10.2105/ajph.2011.300193.

48. Van de Ven AH, Poole MS. Methods for studying innovation development in the Minnesota Innovation Research Program. *Organ Sci* 1990; 1: 313–35. www.jstor.org/stable/2635008 (accessed 10 November 2020).

49. Van de Ven AH. *The Innovation Journey*. Oxford: Oxford University Press; 1999. https://books.google.co.uk/books?id=9nu2zQEACAAJ (accessed 22 January 2023).

50. Checkland K, Harrison S, Marshall M. Is the metaphor of 'barriers to change' useful in understanding implementation? Evidence from general medical practice. *J Health Serv Res Policy* 2007; 12: 95–100. https://doi.org/10.1258/135581907780279657.

51. Langley A, Denis J-L. Beyond evidence: The micropolitics of improvement. *BMJ Qual Saf* 2011; 20: i43–i46. https://doi.org/10.1136/bmjqs.2010.046482.

52. Martin G, Dixon-Woods M. Collaboration-based approaches. In: Dixon-Woods M, Brown K, Marjanovic S, et al., editors. *Elements of Improving Quality and Safety in Healthcare*. Cambridge: Cambridge University Press; 2022. https://doi.org/10.1017/9781009236867.

53. Carter P, Ozieranski P, McNicol S, Power M, Dixon-Woods M. How collaborative are quality improvement collaboratives: A qualitative study in stroke care. *Implement Sci* 2014; 9: 32. https://doi.org/10.1186/1748-5908-9-32.

54. Rashman L, Hartley J. Leading and learning? Knowledge transfer in the Beacon Council Scheme. *Public Administration* 2002; 80: 523–42. https://doi.org/10.1111/1467-9299.00316.

55. Lennox L, Linwood-Amor A, Maher L, Reed J. Making change last? Exploring the value of sustainability approaches in healthcare: A scoping

review. *Health Res Policy Syst* 2020; 18: 120. https://doi.org/10.1186/s12961-020-00601-0.

56. Massoud M, Nielsen G, Nolan K, et al. *A Framework for Spread: From Local Improvements to System-wide Change.* Cambridge, MA: Institute for Healthcare Improvement; 2006. www.ihi.org/resources/Pages/IHIWhitePapers/AFrameworkforSpreadWhitePaper.aspx (accessed 22 January 2023).

57. Slaghuis SS, Strating MMH, Bal RA, Nieboer AP. A framework and a measurement instrument for sustainability of work practices in long-term care. *BMC Health Serv Res* 2011; 11: 314. https://doi.org/10.1186/1472-6963-11-314.

58. Urquhart R, Kendell C, Cornelissen E, et al. Identifying factors influencing sustainability of innovations in cancer survivorship care: A qualitative study. *BMJ Open* 2021; 11: e042503. https://doi.org/10.1136/bmjopen-2020-042503.

59. Jeffs L, Jamieson T, Saragosa M, et al. Uptake and scalability of a peritoneal dialysis virtual care solution: Qualitative study. *JMIR Hum Factors* 2019; 6: e9720. https://doi.org/10.2196/humanfactors.9720.

60. Weiss D, Kassam-Adams N, Murray C, et al. Application of a framework to implement trauma-informed care throughout a pediatric health care network. *J Contin Educ Health Prof* 2017; 37: 55–60. https://doi.org/10.1097/CEH.0000000000000140.

61. Greenhalgh T, Wherton J, Papoutsi C, et al. Analysing the role of complexity in explaining the fortunes of technology programmes: Empirical application of the NASSS framework. *BMC Med* 2018; 16: 66. https://doi.org/10.1186/s12916-018-1050-6.

62. Papoutsi C, A'Court C, Wherton J, Shaw S, Greenhalgh T. Explaining the mixed findings of a randomised controlled trial of telehealth with centralised remote support for heart failure: Multi-site qualitative study using the NASSS framework. *Trials* 2020; 21: 891. https://doi.org/10.1186/s13063-020-04817-x.

63. Doyle C, Howe C, Woodcock T, et al. Making change last: Applying the NHS institute for innovation and improvement sustainability model to healthcare improvement. *Implement Sci* 2013; 8: 1–10. https://doi.org/10.1186/1748-5908-8-127.

64. Van Oppen JD, Thompson D, Tite M, et al. The Acute Frailty Network: Experiences from a whole-systems quality improvement collaborative for acutely ill older patients in the English NHS. *Eur Geriatr Med* 2019; 10: 559–65. https://doi.org/10.1007/s41999-019-00177-1.

65. May C, Finch T. Implementing, embedding, and integrating practices: An outline of normalization process theory. *Sociology* 2009; 43: 535–54. https://doi.org/10.1177/0038038509103208.

66. Pope C, Halford S, Turnbull J, et al. Using computer decision support systems in NHS emergency and urgent care: Ethnographic study using normalisation process theory. *BMC Health Serv Res* 2013; 13: 1–13. https://doi.org/10.1186/1472-6963-13-111.

67. Murray E, Treweek S, Pope C, et al. Normalisation process theory: A framework for developing, evaluating and implementing complex interventions. *BMC Med* 2010; 8: 1–11. https://doi.org/10.1186/1741-7015-8-63.

68. Cramm JM, Nieboer AP. Short and long term improvements in quality of chronic care delivery predict program sustainability. *Soc Sci Med* 2014; 101: 148–54. https://doi.org/10.1016/j.socscimed.2013.11.035.

69. Stolldorf DP. Sustaining health care interventions to achieve quality care: What we can learn from rapid response teams. *J Nurs Care Qual* 2017; 32: 87–93. https://doi.org/10.1097/NCQ.0000000000000204.

70. Ghiron L, Shillingi L, Kabiswa C, et al. Beginning with sustainable scale up in mind: Initial results from a population, health and environment project in East Africa. *Reprod Health Matters* 2014; 22: 84–92. https://doi.org/10.1016/S0968-8080(14)43761-3.

71. Geels FW. The multi-level perspective on sustainability transitions: Responses to seven criticisms. *Environ Innov Soc Transit* 2011; 1: 24–40. https://doi.org/10.1016/j.eist.2011.02.002.

72. Geels FW, Kern F, Fuchs G, et al. The enactment of socio-technical transition pathways: A reformulated typology and a comparative multi-level analysis of the German and UK low-carbon electricity transitions (1990–2014). *Res Pol* 2016; 45: 896–913. https://doi.org/10.1016/j.respol.2016.01.015.

73. Marjanovic S, Altenhofer M, Hocking L, Chataway J, Ling T. Innovating for improved healthcare: Sociotechnical and innovation systems perspectives and lessons from the NHS. *Sci Public Policy* 2020; 47: 283–97. https://doi.org/10.1093/scipol/scaa005.

74. Flynn R, Mrklas K, Campbell A, Wasylak T, Scott SD. Contextual factors and mechanisms that influence sustainability: A realist evaluation of two scaled, multi-component interventions. *BMC Health Serv Res* 2021; 21: 1194. https://doi.org/10.1186/s12913-021-07214-5.

75. Austin EE, Blakely B, Salmon P, Braithwaite J, Clay-Williams R. Technology in the emergency department: Using cognitive work analysis

to model and design sustainable systems. *Saf Sci* 2022; 147: 105613. https://doi.org/10.1016/j.ssci.2021.105613.

76. Øvretveit J, Staines A. Sustained improvement? Findings from an independent case study of the Jönköping quality program. *Qual Manage Healthcare* 2007; 16: 68–83. https://doi.org/10.1097/00019514-200701000-00009.

77. Øvretveit J. Widespread focused improvement: Lessons from international health for spreading specific improvements to health services in high-income countries. *Int J Qual Health Care* 2011; 23: 239–46. https://doi.org/10.1093/intqhc/mzr018.

78. Greenhalgh T, Maylor H, Shaw S, et al. The NASSS-CAT tools for understanding, guiding, monitoring, and researching technology implementation projects in health and social care: Protocol for an evaluation study in real-world settings. *JMIR Res Protoc* 2020; 9: e16861. https://doi.org/10.2196/16861.

79. Abimbola S, Patel B, Peiris D, et al. The NASSS framework for ex post theorisation of technology-supported change in healthcare: Worked example of the TORPEDO programme. *BMC Med* 2019; 17: 233. https://doi.org/10.1186/s12916-019-1463-x.

80. Nuffield Department of Primary Care Health Sciences. *What Are the NASSS-CAT Tools?* Oxford: Nuffield Department of Primary Care Health Sciences; 2022. www.phc.ox.ac.uk/research/interdisciplinary-research-in-health-sciences/enasss-cat (accessed 22 January 2023).

81. The PROMPT Maternity Foundation. What is PROMPT? www.promptmaternity.org (accessed 22 January 2023).

82. Crofts J, Ellis D, Draycott T, et al. Change in knowledge of midwives and obstetricians following obstetric emergency training: A randomised controlled trial of local hospital, simulation centre and teamwork training. *BJOG* 2007; 114: 1534–41. https://doi.org/10.1111/j.1471-0528.2007.01493.x.

83. Draycott T, Winter C. Interviewed by: Marjanovic S. Interview on Spread and Scale-Up of an Obstetric Emergency Training Package with Professor Tim Draycott, Consultant Obstetrician at North Bristol NHS Trust, and Dr Cathy Winter, Senior Midwife at North Bristol Trust & Lead Midwife for the PROMPT Maternity Foundation. [Personal interview, 26 March] 2020 (unpublished).

84. Draycott T. *Practical Obstetric Multi-professional Training*. London: The Health Foundation; 2013. https://improve.bmj.com/sites/default/files/resources/prompt.pdf (accessed 22 January 2023).

85. Draycott T, Sibanda T, Owen L, et al. Does training in obstetric emergencies improve neonatal outcome? *BJOG* 2006; 113: 177–82. https://doi.org/10.1111/j.1471-0528.2006.00800.x.

86. Draycott TJ, Crofts JF, Ash JP, et al. Improving neonatal outcome through practical shoulder dystocia training. *Obstet Gynecol* 2008; 112: 14–20. https://doi.org/10.1097/AOG.0b013e31817bbc61.

87. The PROMPT Foundation. PROMPT's story. www.promptmaternity.org/prompt-uk-1 (accessed 22 January 2023).

88. Crofts J, Lenguerrand E, Bentham G, et al. Prevention of brachial plexus injury – 12 years of shoulder dystocia training: An interrupted time-series study. *BJOG* 2016; 123: 111–8. https://doi.org/10.1111/1471-0528.13302.

89. Lenguerrand E, Winter C, Innes K, et al. THISTLE: Trial of hands-on interprofessional simulation training for local emergencies: A research protocol for a stepped-wedge clustered randomised controlled trial. *BMC Pregnancy Childbirth* 2017; 17: 1–9. https://doi.org/10.1186/s12884-017-1455-9.

90. Renwick S, Hookes S, Draycott T, et al. PROMPT Wales project: National scaling of an evidence-based intervention to improve safety and training in maternity. *BMJ Open Qual* 2021; 10: e001280. https://doi.org/10.1136/bmjoq-2020-001280.

91. Offord N, Wyrko Z, Downes T, et al. Frailsafe: From conception to national breakthrough collaborative. *Acute Med* 2016; 15(3): 109–64. https://doi.org/10.52964/AMJA.0624.

92. Institute for Healthcare Improvement. The breakthrough series: IHI's collaborative model for achieving breakthrough improvement. *Diabetes Spectr* 2004; 17: 97–101. https://doi.org/10.2337/diaspect.17.2.97.

93. Papoutsi C, Poots A, Clements J, et al. Improving patient safety for older people in acute admissions: Implementation of the Frailsafe checklist in 12 hospitals across the UK. *Age and Ageing* 2018; 47: 311–7. https://doi.org/10.1093/ageing/afx194.

94. Lanham HJ, Leykum LK, Taylor BS, et al. How complexity science can inform scale-up and spread in health care: Understanding the role of self-organization in variation across local contexts. *Soc Sci Med* 2013; 93: 194–202. https://doi.org/10.1016/j.socscimed.2012.05.040.

95. Ali G-C, Altenhofer M, Gloinson ER, Marjanovic S. *What Influences Improvement Processes in Healthcare? A Rapid Evidence Review.* Santa Monica, CA: RAND Corporation; 2020. www.rand.org/pubs/research_reports/RRA440-1.html (accessed 22 January 2023).

96. Robert G, Locock L, Williams O, et al. Co-producing and co-designing. In: Dixon-Woods M, Brown K, Marjanovic S, et al., editors. *Elements of*

Improving Quality and Safety in Healthcare. Cambridge: Cambridge University Press; 2022. https://doi.org/10.1017/9781009237024.

97. Sturke R, Vorkoper S, Bekker L-G, et al. Fostering successful and sustainable collaborations to advance implementation science: The adolescent HIV prevention and treatment implementation science alliance. *J Int AIDS Soc* 2020; 23: e25572. https://doi.org/10.1002/jia2.25572.

98. Spicer N, Bhattacharya D, Dimka R, et al. 'Scaling-up is a craft not a science': Catalysing scale-up of health innovations in Ethiopia, India and Nigeria. *Soc Sci Med* 2014; 121: 30–8. https://doi.org/10.1016/j.socscimed.2014.09.046.

99. NHS England. Leading the spread and adoption of innovation andimprovement: A practical guide. www.england.nhs.uk/spread-and-adoption (accessed 22 January 2023).

Cambridge Elements ⊒

Improving Quality and Safety in Healthcare

Editors-in-Chief

Mary Dixon-Woods

THIS Institute (The Healthcare Improvement Studies Institute)

Mary is Director of THIS Institute and is the Health Foundation Professor of Healthcare Improvement Studies in the Department of Public Health and Primary Care at the University of Cambridge. Mary leads a programme of research focused on healthcare improvement, healthcare ethics, and methodological innovation in studying healthcare.

Graham Martin

THIS Institute (The Healthcare Improvement Studies Institute)

Graham is Director of Research at THIS Institute, leading applied research programmes and contributing to the institute's strategy and development. His research interests are in the organisation and delivery of healthcare, and particularly the role of professionals, managers, and patients and the public in efforts at organisational change.

Executive Editor

Katrina Brown

THIS Institute (The Healthcare Improvement Studies Institute)

Katrina is Communications Manager at THIS Institute, providing editorial expertise to maximise the impact of THIS Institute's research findings. She managed the project to produce the series.

Editorial Team

Sonja Marjanovic

RAND Europe

Sonja is Director of RAND Europe's healthcare innovation, industry, and policy research. Her work provides decision-makers with evidence and insights to support innovation and improvement in healthcare systems, and to support the translation of innovation into societal benefits for healthcare services and population health.

Tom Ling

RAND Europe

Tom is Head of Evaluation at RAND Europe and President of the European Evaluation Society, leading evaluations and applied research focused on the key challenges facing health services. His current health portfolio includes evaluations of the innovation landscape, quality improvement, communities of practice, patient flow, and service transformation.

Ellen Perry

THIS Institute (The Healthcare Improvement Studies Institute)

Ellen supported the production of the series during 2020–21.

About the Series

The past decade has seen enormous growth in both activity and research on improvement in healthcare. This series offers a comprehensive and authoritative set of overviews of the different improvement approaches available, exploring the thinking behind them, examining evidence for each approach, and identifying areas of debate.

Cambridge Elements ⁼

Improving Quality and Safety in Healthcare

Elements in the Series

Collaboration-Based Approaches
Graham Martin and Mary Dixon-Woods

Co-Producing and Co-Designing
Glenn Robert, Louise Locock, Oli Williams, Jocelyn Cornwell, Sara Donetto,
and Joanna Goodrich

The Positive Deviance Approach
Ruth Baxter and Rebecca Lawton

Implementation Science
Paul Wilson and Roman Kislov

Making Culture Change Happen
Russell Mannion

Operational Research Approaches
Martin Utley, Sonya Crowe, and Christina Pagel

Reducing Overuse
Caroline Cupit, Carolyn Tarrant, and Natalie Armstrong

Simulation as an Improvement Technique
Victoria Brazil, Eve Purdy, and Komal Bajaj

Workplace Conditions
Jill Maben, Jane Ball, and Amy C. Edmondson

Governance and Leadership
Naomi J. Fulop and Angus I. G. Ramsay

Health Economics
Andrew Street and Nils Gutacker

Approaches to Spread, Scale-Up, and Sustainability
Chrysanthi Papoutsi, Trisha Greenhalgh, and Sonja Marjanovic

Printed in the United States
by Baker & Taylor Publisher Services